Medicinal Herbs:
20 Healing Herbs and Herbal Mixes

Table of content

Introduction: The Best Things Come from Scratch! 3

Chapter 1: Aromatherapy; A Nose above the Rest! 5

Chapter 2: Healing Through Essential Oils 11

Chapter 3: The Herbal Medicine Cabinet 16

Chapter 4: Herbal Aids for Weight Loss 23

Chapter 5: Herbs for Health, Beauty, and Cosmetics...27

Conclusion: Staying Healthy For Life...30

FREE Bonus Reminder...31

Introduction: The Best Things Come from Scratch!

About as far back as conscious, human recollection goes, herbs from man's natural environment have been used for medicinal purposes. They were used in India over 5000 years ago in the form of Ayurvedic Medicine. And in ancient Greece, for a physician named Aristotle, the power of flowers, fruits, seeds and roots, was just what the doctor ordered.

Herbal medicine was the standard form of treatment for much of the world for centuries. In the past when someone was sick they would pay a visit to their local herbal expert who would find just the right ingredient to help them. A sorely missed ingredient for most of us in modern life, since in much of the prepackaged and mass produced modern world, we are hard pressed to even find herbs in the food we eat, let alone are medicine. But as this book bears testament—things are starting to change!

And herbal therapies are starting to make a major come back. And one of the most popular herbal therapies to make some headway is that of Aromatherapy. With its roots firmly affixed to the incense burners of the ancient world, this herbal practice has us purposefully inhaling the fragrance of specific herbs in order to create a desired reaction in our body. A powerful treatment that has now sprung up as special Aromatherapy clinics attached to many major hospitals.

In recent years the use of taking he essential oils from medicinal herbs and using them in specifically targeted massage therapy has also become in vogue. We will discuss both of these practices and many more methods further in this book. For right now I just want to captivate your imagination with the possibilities and ignite your awareness of the impact that these powerful medicinal herbs can have on your life.

Sometimes known as holistic medicine, medicinal herbs are used to treat the whole body. This holistic approach is something that modern medicine often lacks. Because often enough, when we turn to pharmaceuticals we find ourselves just masking chronic symptoms, whereas many herbal medicines are able to target the actual deficiency itself, which is the source of the problem. Showing once again that, most of our aches and pains are simply our body crying out for something that it lacks.

Because when you break it all down, just as the Christian/Hebrew bible and many other ancient religious traditions remind us; we came from the dust of the Earth. We truly are part and parcel to this planet, and all of the molecules, all of the proteins, amino acids and other trace elements in our body can be found strewn all over the Earth. So if this is from whence we came, and we find that our body is lacking something, all we have to do is look to the Earth to find it. We don't need to replicate and synthesize chemicals in a pharmacy; all we have to do is look to nature and the medicines that it naturally provides. Because the best things truly do come from scratch!

Chapter 1: Aromatherapy; A Nose above the Rest!

The human nose is an intricate piece of sensory machinery, we may not be aware of the complexities involved in smelling a cup of coffee, but that doesn't mean that they are not there. Called the "Chemosensory System" the nose is part of a joint apparatus that works to use the senses of taste and smell in order to help us interpret our environment.

For thousands of years our sense of smell has served to help us find a meal, tell us of potential threats, and through pheromones that trigger powerful chemosensory responses, has even played a role in determining our mates. We may take it for granted and not realize how influential are noses are, but just try to go a few days without it and you will quickly realize what you are missing.

Our noses work hard to interpret our environment, constantly labeling and cataloging a vast multitude of chemical molecules that we inhale every time we breathe in the air. In an instant our nose is able to pick up the distinct chemical trace element of a campfire and then send it to our brain which instantly relates to us our fond memories of when we used to go camping with our Uncle Bernie.

Every time we smell a specific "smell" it is due to the fact that an odor molecule has bonded to one of the millions of "olfactory receptors" in our nasal cavity whose job is to interpret what those odor molecules are. Telling us whether something is bitter, salty, sweet, or one of a million variations in between. These incredibly complex interchanges happen in an instant—and faster than you can say, "This stinks!"—your nose is way ahead of you relaying that information!

As you can see, the nose is on the front line of our senses and working as a great interpreter of what is good for us, and what is not so good for us in the chemical makeup of our world. The nose also works as a natural gateway when it comes to the field of herbal medicine. It was also the original "gateway drug" in ancient religious practice in which incense was a common feature of inducing more mindful states for ceremonies and to relieve the stress of participants.

Frankincense

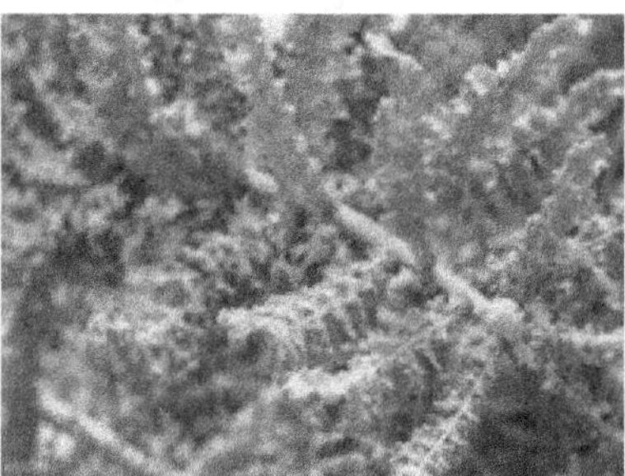

Powerful herbs were burned by the boatload in order to set the mood of the faithful. Smelling powerful incense was always a powerful part of religious service, making medicinal herbs a highly prized possession. And one of the most famous of these herbs is that of "Frankincense". Who could forget this wonder drug of the ancients? This was a medicinal herb that was so spectacular that it even made a cameo in the first Christmas story. Does anyone remember the three Magi who carried their Frankincense and Myrrh all the way from Persia?

In ancient times this stuff was of such high value that it was sometimes doled out as its own kind of currency. Frankincense was known to be able to alter the chemistry of the brain just by inhaling its fragrance. When the ancients were feeling a bit down in the doldrums they would just burn incense laced with Frankincense for an all natural herbal pick-me-up. And besides the elevation of mood it was discovered to have great affect on treating many kinds of inflammation.

It was quite a common practice for the local apothecary of yesteryear to either massage a bit of Frankincense into their patient's aching joints, or to have them just take a deep breath of their burning Frankincense cauldrons. Because just the smell of Frankincense alone can kick start a powerful chemical reaction in the body that cleanses it from impurities and boosts the immune system.

In modern day Ayurvedic circles Frankincense has even been known to fight cancer. Studies have shown that the application of Frankincense can reduce the onset or even reverse the incidence of Basil Cell Carcinoma (Skin Cancer), demonstrating exactly why this medicinal herb continues to be such a valuable commodity to this very day. Just by taking a breath of fresh air we can revitalize our entire system.

This is the basic premise that aromatherapy has been based on. But besides incense, one of the other traditional ways to take in the fragrance of medicinal herbs is to make an old fashioned poultice. A poultice is a distribution method of directly applying herbs to the skin, often around the neck and shoulders, so that the aroma of the herbs can be directly inhaled over a long period of time.

Poultices usually consist of dried out plant material rather than liquid and are crushed or mashed together and boiled with water before their application in order to make the ingredients more malleable so they can be easily pasted onto the skin. The poultice is often held onto the chest or neck area as a compress, fixed in place with heavy gauze.

Chamomile

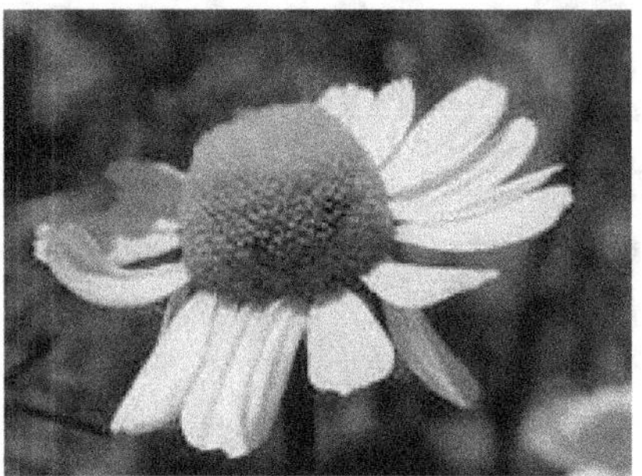

The herb Chamomile which is most famously known for its properties in tea also doubles as a great poultice. The crushed petals of the Chamomile flower compressed over a bruise or area of severe inflammation can bring immediate relief through this powerful poultice. The Chamomile poultice is also effective when placed on the jaw to relieve toothaches or around the ear to relieve a bad earache. But as mentioned you don't have to wear a poultice to get the effects of Chamomile.

Because a good strong blend of Chamomile tea can do wonders to alleviate muscle aches, as well as improve symptoms of anxiety and depression. And along with relaxing our nerves, breathing in the aroma of Chamomile has also been shown to relax our blood vessels, helping us to keep our blood pressure under control.

In order to get a good whiff of tea variety Chamomile make yourself a steaming hot mug and pour the tea into the mug hot. And before you even drink it, just put your face close and cup your hands around the mug and your nose, letting yourself breathe in deep the aroma of your tea. You can also just pull up a chair to your tea kettle and simply sit by the stove breathing in the steady aroma steaming out of your tea pot. Either way the effect is the same.

Bergamot

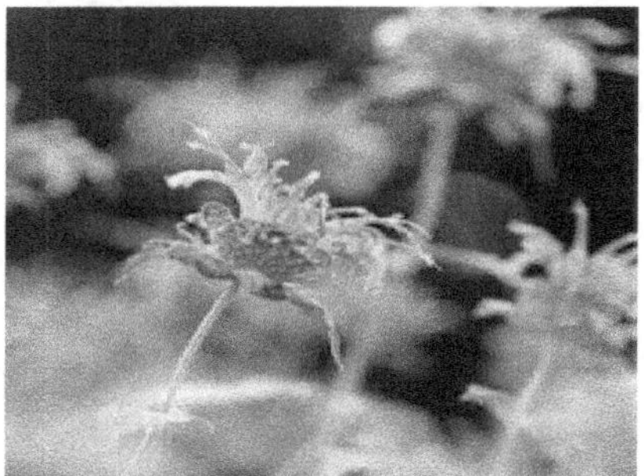

Very similar to the effects of Chamomile, is that of Bergamot, another relaxation inducing herb that can be used in either incense, a poultice wrap or in a great tasting cup of tea. Along with aiding relaxation, Bergamot has some other additional medicinal properties completely unique to this herb. With one of them being its amazing propensity to enable the body to completely neutralize the effects of fevers. Bergamot also works as a powerful disinfectant and antioxidant.

Due to its notable healing properties with the skin this herbal remedy is often taken with a bath either by placing a few drops of Bergamot essential oil (we will discuss essential oils further in the next chapter) or by specially manufactured soaps that have the Bergamot baked right in. Either way, with all of these powerful aromatic options, you will be head and shoulders (and head and nose) above the rest!

Chapter 2: Healing Through Essential Oils

Essential Oils are basically a refined gathering of plant based matter in liquid form. Inside this broad grouping of gathered plant material, we can break Essential Oils down into 8 main categories. They are; floral, citrus, herbaceous, spicy, resinous, earthy, and camphoraceous. All of these categories of Essential Oils are known to serve different purposes. But probably the most widely used however, are those that are derived from the floral family of essential oils.

Rose

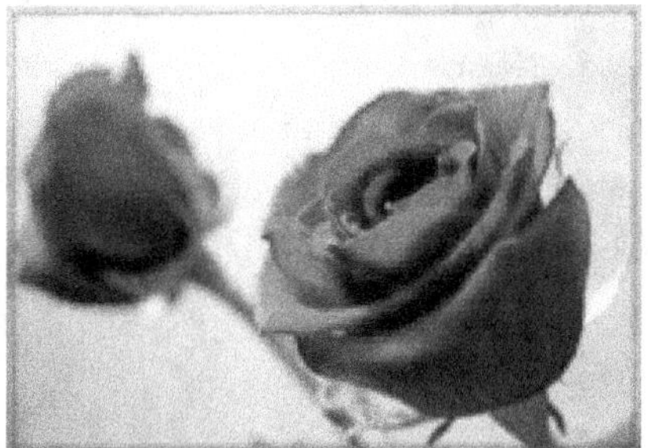

You don't have to look much farther than the expression, "It's time to stop and smell the roses." To realize just how widespread our attachment to floral fauna is. Roses in particular have been known to have many positive medicinal effects on the human body. For example, the petals from a rose when ground into essential oil have been known to be able to treat insomnia, stress, and depression. It has also been widely reported to be able to work as an anti-viral agent that helps boost the immune system.

Geranium

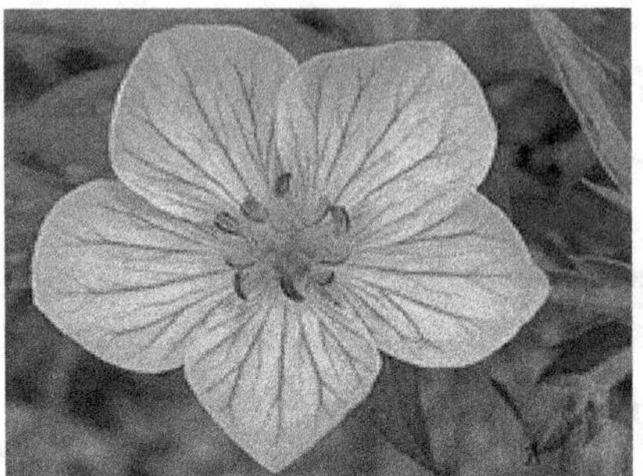

But as good as the rose is, it is also a costly herbal remedy, so much so, that many have opted to use its closest cousin instead. Because the oil derived from the Geranium is known to be nearly identical to oil derived from roses. Its benefits are also very similar, like roses the Geranium is known to have an immediate stress relieving quality when used in aromatherapy or when the oil is massaged into the skin.

Just like the roses, this essential oil also has powerful anti-viral and immune system boosting properties. Geranium oil also works extraordinarily well as a treatment for some of the side effects that women experience during their menstrual cycle as well as helping to alleviate the symptoms of menopause. Another reason that many women swear by this essential oil is also due to its widely known ability to reduce stretch marks which of course is a welcome relief after pregnancy.

But whether it is used for men or women, the compounds found in Geranium essential oil have been known to be able to completely balance out our hormones and help us function on a more even keel. Germanium as a relaxing agent helps to make our muscles contract, it aids our blood vessels in their constriction, and even works to loosen up digestive systems that are plagued with indigestion.

The other interesting thing about Geranium oil is that it is what we call in the world of aromatherapy, a "circulatory oil". This means that rather than releasing the chemical compounds directly upon exhalation—as is the case with other fragrances—the inhalation of Geranium sticks with us and instead of leaving when we breathe out, it goes straight to our blood where it continues to circulate in the body.

But even though we don't exhale the molecules out, they do have to leave the body eventually, and it is the method in which Geranium leaves us that creates another pleasant side effect. Geranium essential oil can only leave us when it is sweated out of the skin. Turning the user of this substance into a living, breathing air freshener, emitting the attractive scent of Geranium just from perspiring! This can have many medicinal uses for someone if they suffer from excessive body odor and it has been known to work as a treatment due to its great deodorizing effects.

<u>*Lotus*</u>

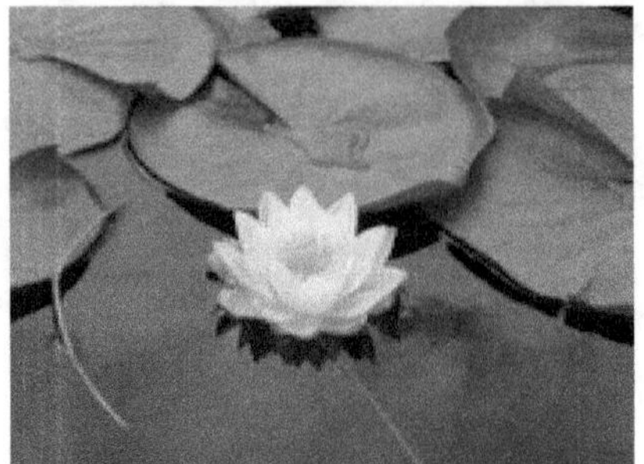

But probably one of the most celebrated oils to ever be extracted from a medicinal herb is that of Lotus oil. Known in the Eastern Hemisphere for thousands of years, the lotus blossom has been the stuff of legend. Along with countless Indian Yogi's down through the centuries, it is said that Buddha himself had prescribed this medicinal herb to his followers, making this medicinal herb a hallmark of two major religions.

But it is the essential oil extracted from this plant that can really create some mind blowing effects. Because just a little bit of lotus oil opens up the lungs and induces a feeling of calm. It would seem to be no coincidence then that the "lotus position" that has become so synonymous with Buddhism and meditation is associated with this flower. The lotus and its oil can have a major impact on our feelings of well being.

Jasmine

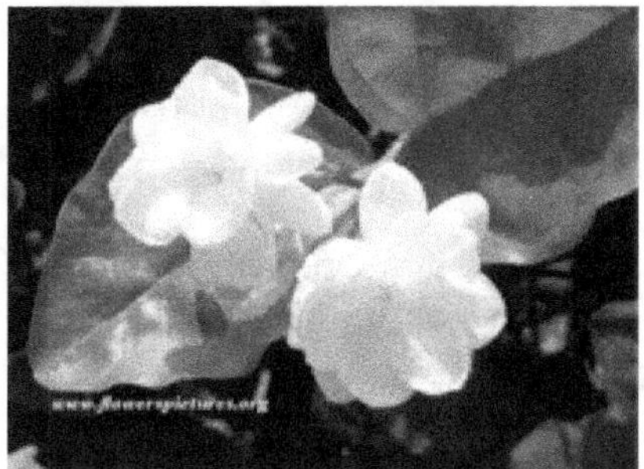

Right next to the effects of the oil from the Lotus, Jasmine essential oil is also a powerful medicinal herb in its own right. Coming from a flower that carries the moniker of "King of Flowers" the scent of Jasmine is unmistakable. I can testify about this from my own personal experience because years ago my senses were frequently inundated with this lovely sent in the most unlikely of places.

When I was still in college I used to do payroll for a truck company and right outside the door to our office someone had planted a ton of these Jasmine flowers and every spring when the flowers bloomed, we were all overwhelmed with their powerful scent. And whoever walked in the door when these flowers were nearby seemed to instantly perk up to their fragrance.

Even the big burly truck drivers who were on layover at our facility seemed to become rather pleasant and tranquil with this aroma around. Showing that even the toughest and gruffest of truck drivers need to take the time to smell the roses! Yet another example of just how soothing and medicinal the essential oils from these herbs can be; providing a bit of healing for us all.

Chapter 3: The Herbal Medicine Cabinet

Most of the time we are always hearing about the "latest" advances in medicine and high tech methods to treat illnesses. But what about some of the low tech options such as medicinal herbs that have been with us for thousands of years?

Because no matter what you may be up against, whatever sickness or ailment that you may be facing the immense bounty of nature and its medicinal herbs is bound to have the solution you are looking for. So let's stock up our low tech medicine cabinet on some of the most important medicinal herbs for daily health, as well as emergencies.

Echinacea

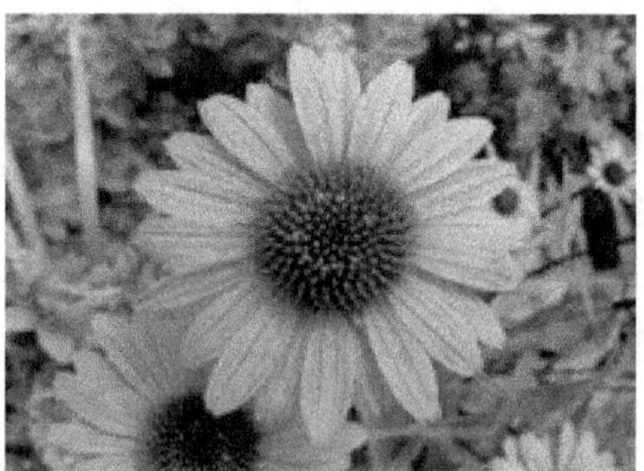

The first addition to our herbal medicine cabinet has been used by Native Americans for years for its anti-viral and anti-biotic properties. Echinacea is a potent herb and when ground into powder or the oil is extracted it is a powerful fighting agent against germs, viruses, bacteria, and even warts! So be sure to stock your herbal medicine cabinet with this precious resource.

Aloe Vera

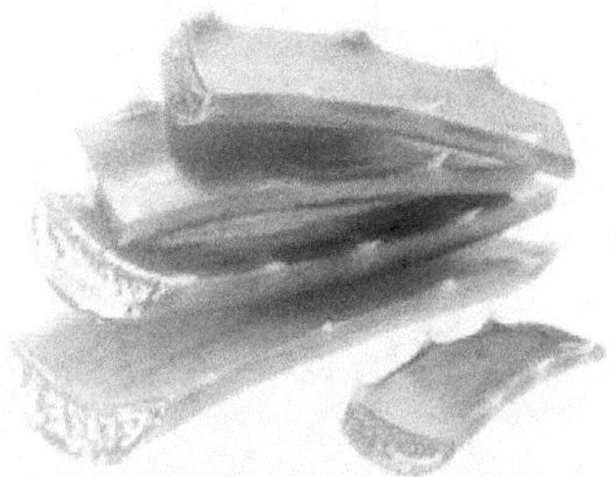

Growing up in Florida, as a child I learned from first hand experience that if you live in an environment with a lot of sunshine then Aloe Vera can be your best friend. Aloe Vera has been used to treat sunburns for a long time and is fast becoming standard fare even in burn units at hospitals. So if you are out in the sun and wind up with a bad burn it could help you out quite a bit if you have some of this stuff on hand.

Nowadays this Aloe Vera is fairly ubiquitous and you can find it at just about any CVS or Walgreens drugstore, but you don't have to buy it, because you can always just make your own. I'm a big fan of DIY and truly believe in the mantra that if you can do it yourself; then you might as well do it!

In order to make your own Aloe Vera you will need a leaf from the Aloe Vera Plant, the leaves of this plant are naturally full of the very same gel that you would buy at the drug store. So just take a leaf off this plant and either break it or cut it with a knife or scissors and squeeze the gel out into a small bowl.

After you've squeezed the gel into your bowl you can go ahead and scoop it out with a spoon or your fingers and apply it directly to your skin. Or if you would like to save it for later simply cover the bowl and put it in a cool and dry place such as a cabinet or possibly a first aid kit.

Catnip

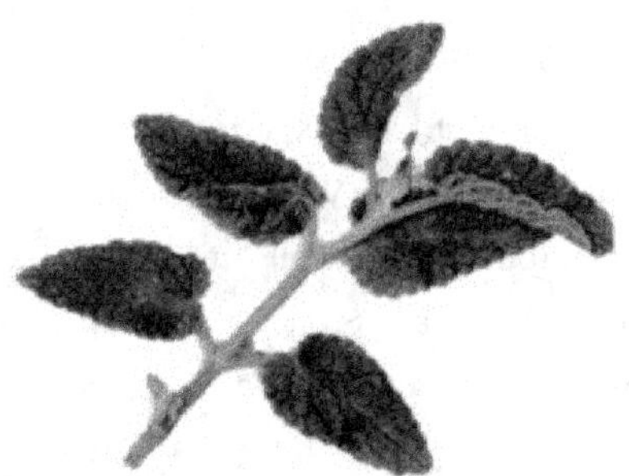

Our next recommendation for your low tech medicine cabinet is probably going to come as a bit of a surprise (for you and your cat) because as it turns out, catnip has many medicinal properties beyond making your feline friends go berserk. Catnip when used properly (for humans) is a natural cure for insomnia. Ground up leaves from the Catnip plant can be used to make medicinal teas that help sooth and relax those who drink them..

This same relaxing effect is also known to relax the digestive system, so if you are having stomach issues drinking a relaxing blend of catnip tea may be just the thing to put your troubled stomach at ease. It's also been well documented in its ability to help relieve headaches, so whether you are having trouble with your nerves, your sleep, your stomach or just have a nasty migraine, a medicinal blend of this catnip herb just might help you out.

Mistletoe

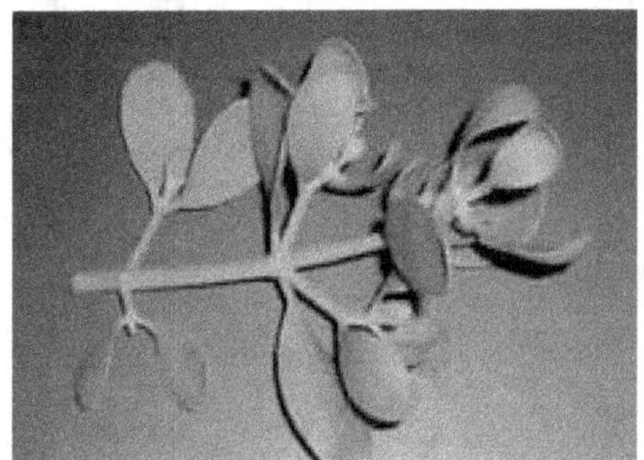

Another medicinal herb you may be surprised to find as a must have in your Herbal Medicine Cabinet is that of the most notorious hanger-on the holiday season has ever known; the Mistletoe. Yes, yes, I know you are probably rolling your eyes as you fight to keep "Ho, Ho, the Mistletoe!" from becoming stuck in your head, but please hear me out. Because this thing has a medicinal worth that goes far beyond holiday smooching.

For a plant that has such loving connotations, the Mistletoe's origins are actually that of a parasite. Normally found attached to Oak and Hawthorn trees, the Mistletoe receives its nourishment by leeching onto other plants. The great thing the Mistletoe does when it attaches itself to the nervous system of humans however, is that it has been found to be a wonderful anti-spasmodic agent that works well in treating convulsive nervous disorders such as epilepsy.

The leaves of this plant have been valued for quite a long time as a nervine and antispasmodic herbal medicine. In the past Mistletoe leaves have even been used to treat hysteria. Teas from Mistletoe leaves have also been known to help slow down a rapid heart rate, relieve high blood pressure, and soothe aching bones. But a word of caution however, the berries of this plant are mildly toxic and people have been known to get sick from eating them. The berries of the Mistletoe should be left alone; any medicinal properties of this plant should be derived from the leaves.

Garlic

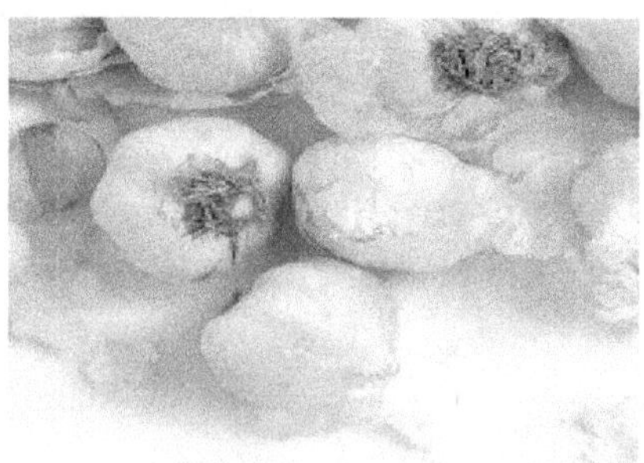

For the next installment in the herbal medicine cabinet we are going to suggest an herbal remedy that can work as an amazing antiseptic and immune booster as well as being rather tasty as a pizza topping. The herb I am talking about is Garlic. Known for its healing properties on the battlefields of the ancient world, crushed cloves of garlic applied directly to cuts and scrapes greatly speeds up the body's ability to heal its wounds.

Garlic is also known to be an incredible immune booster insulating the body well against colds and the flu, making this tasty medicinal herb a definite addition to the herbal medicine cabinet during the cold and flu season. This herb is best in its natural state, so keep a few cloves around that you can grind into powder or boil into your foods.

Astragalus

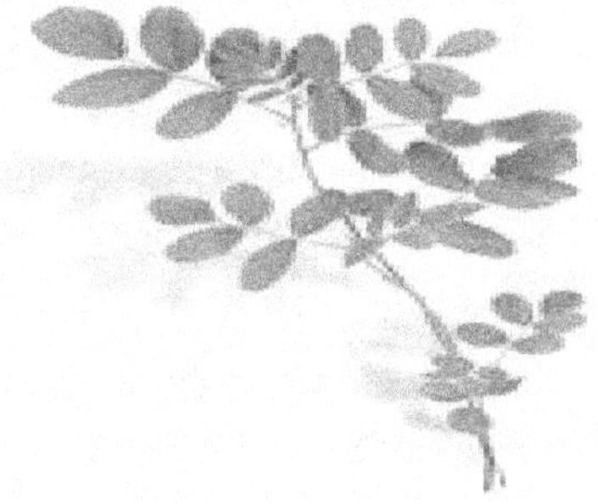

The Chinese herb Astragalus should be another addition to your herbal medicine cabinet. This herb has been used in Chinese medicine for years and is an excellent way to boost the immune system, fight colds, and energize the body. Astragalus is gathered as a root and usually ground into fine powder for use. It can either be applied directly to the skin or boiled in tea.

Dandelion

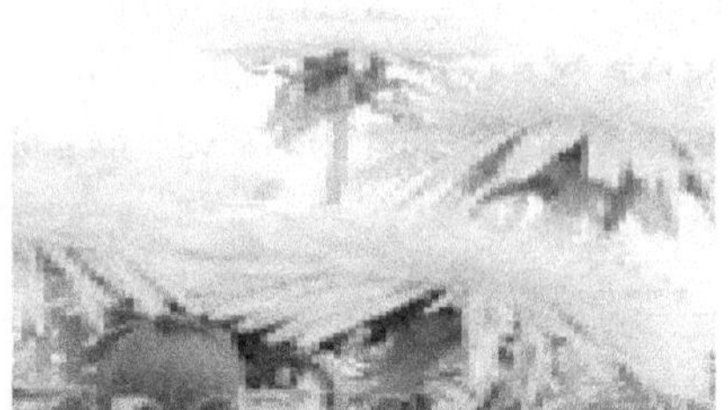

Although this herb is native to Europe it has become quite ubiquitous in North America as well. Known as the "backyard herbal remedy" in a real pinch the Dandelion can be quite useful. Dandelion roots can be drunk as a kind of tonic in teas and even "root" beers. The medicinal benefits of this magical root range from helping to aid indigestion all the way to promoting proper insulin function in diabetics. Providing powerful benefits for your health and making for a great addition to your Herbal Medicine Cabinet.

Chapter 4: Herbal Aids for Weight Loss

With so many people suffering from expanding waist lines, in recent years we are flooded with a never ending litany of dieting fads and gimmicks. Carb restricting regimens such as Atkins and the Paleo diet in particular have become very popular as of late, but the only problem is, once you deviate away from these strict carb reducing regimens the weight comes right back.

The world of herbal medicine when it comes to weight loss has not been immune to criticisms either, as was most famously evidenced from the fallout Dr. Alan Hirsch faced a few years ago over his failed "Sensa" weight loss powder. Do you remember that? Sensa was a supposed aromatherapy based blend of aromatic crystals that people were told to sprinkle over their food to help them lose weight.

The jury still seems to be out on Dr. Hirsch's method, and if it actually worked, but when it comes to whether or not his clients had the right to sue him on false advertising, the jury emphatically agreed in the form of a 26 million dollar lawsuit. But what if we could bypass those mysterious "aromatic crystals" of Sensa and turn to a few proven herbal ingredients to enhance our diet and help to manage our weight the natural way? Look no further than "Rosemary".

Rosemary

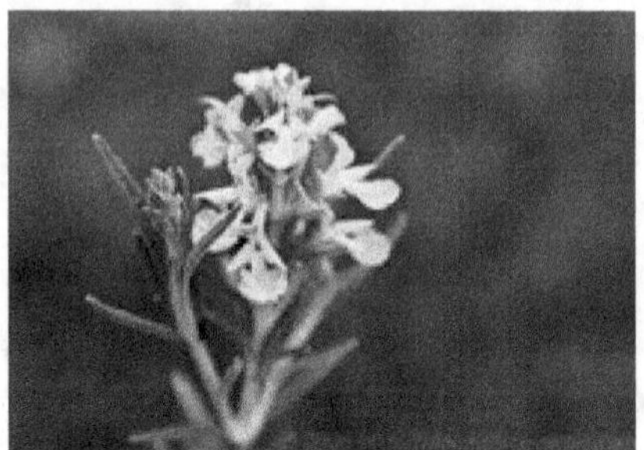

This medicinal herb hails from Asia and has been held in acclaim far and wide for its beneficial properties in regard to regulating weight gain and even eliminating cellulite. When this herb is consumed in a cup of tea it can raise your metabolism helping you to burn fat. Rosemary is also an excellent diuretic and the first weight that this herb will help you lose will undoubtedly be water weight, as this tea directly cleanses your system of excess water and other toxins.

After de-toxing like this, the Rosemary coursing through your system will bring you a new surge of energy and wellness; refreshing you as it cleanses. If you drink this tea for seven days straight your body will be primed, and streamlined with a higher metabolism and completely cleansed of toxins.

Rosemary works to eliminate any previous digestion problems, getting rid of bloating and helping you to break down food faster. As a result you will feel content with your food intake faster, curbing your appetite and keeping you from eating more. Most people lose at least a few pounds after their first weak of exposure to Rosemary and many more claim that this herb has toned their body and eliminated their unsightly cellulite.

Peppermint

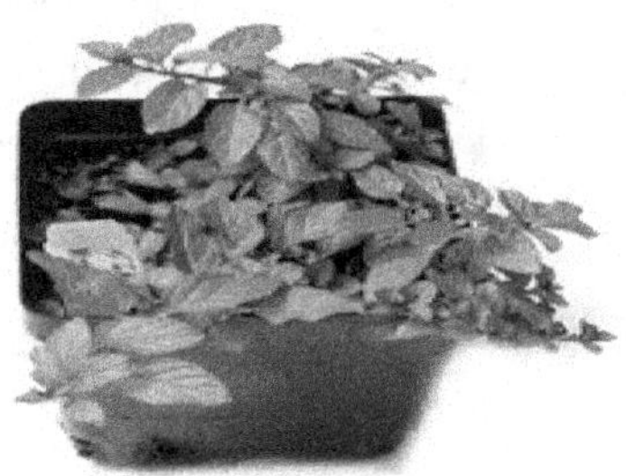

Another good herbal cleanser for the body is peppermint. Peppermint when inhaled and absorbed through the skin can directly influence bile secretion in the digestive tract. An action that helps to suppress appetite and further kick start your metabolism. Peppermint is best burned as incense and inhaled directly or even in a nice warm bath absorbing a diluted amount in your bathwater.

Ginseng

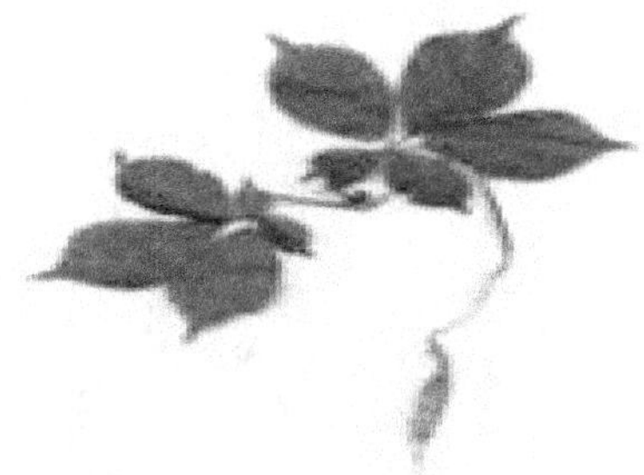

Last but certainly not least in our quest for herbal weight loss is the ancient Chinese herb of Ginseng. The roots from this herb are potent and have been known to boost the metabolism, but much more than this, Ginseng has the uncanny ability to alter the body's cells directly, altering their composition and actually rendering them less capable of storing fat. This herb and all the others mentioned in this chapter are most definitely welcome news for anyone seeking an herbal aid for weight loss.

Chapter 5: Herbs for Health, Beauty, and Cosmetics

Medicinal herbs can be a powerful force of healing in just about every aspect of our lives, beauty and cosmetics is yet another area where these natural remedies can apply. And if you are like 99.9% of the rest of the people on this planet, you probably tend to be a little bit concerned about your hair. Don't worry though because our herbs have us covered in that department as well. Because if you would like to have shiny healthy hair all you need is a few drops of a special little herb called "Sandalwood".

Sandalwood

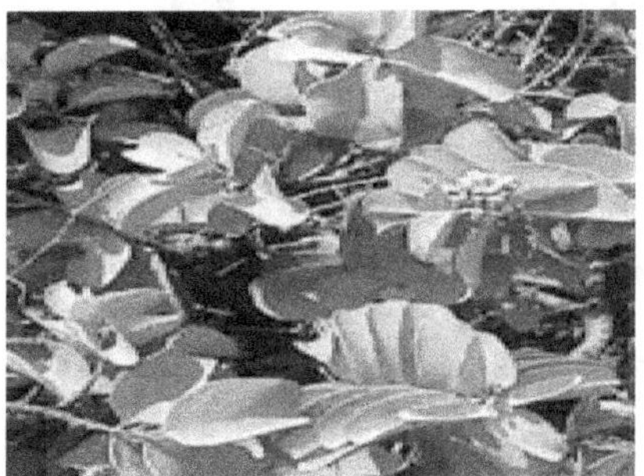

Sandalwood works as a powerful cleansing agent and along with shinier hair, sandalwood does a remarkable job of rejuvenating the skin and enhancing the user's overall complexion. Sandalwood can also work as an active ingredient in relieving the symptoms of Eczema and other skin disorders. Even better for those of us that have already sailed past the age of 30, Sandalwood is known to reduce the appearance of wrinkles. Sandalwood can work its way right under those bags under your eyes, reduce the moisture and make them disappear!

A great homemade mixture for Sandalwood skin cream involves one tablespoon of Sandalwood powder combined with a tablespoon of turmeric in about half a cup of water. Just apply this mixture as a paste to the skin and you will begin to see results right away. Let the paste dry off naturally and you will soon find that your skin has a clear and natural sheen.

Rosewood

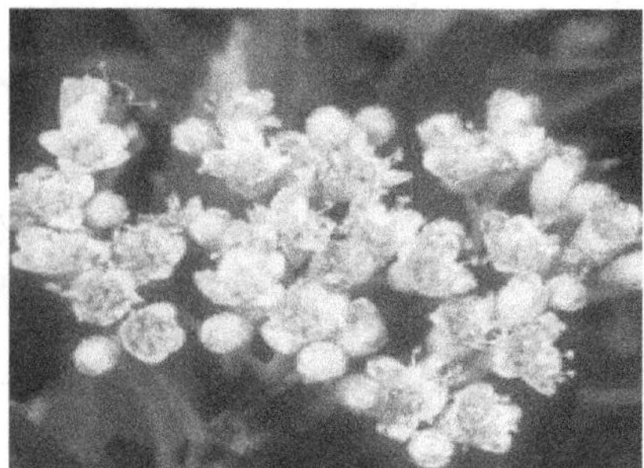

Rosewood is also a great herb for healthy skin and hair, and has been used in soap and shampoo since at least the early 1900's. Rosewood is extracted primarily from trees native to the great rainforests of South America, a fact that has unfortunately led to some pretty bad deforestation. Recent conservation legislation however has fought against this and the extraction of rosewood is highly regulated in order to prevent abuse and unnecessary waste of this precious resource.

<u>Avocado</u>

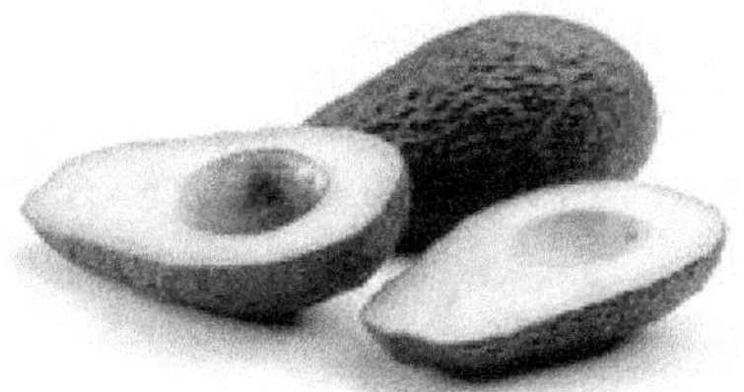

Our next notable mention for cosmetic enhancement you have probably used before to enhance your tacos! I'm talking about Avocados of course! Avocados have long played a role in that familiar face mask that many women (and some men) have ritually went to bed with over the years. It's sometimes remembered more as a running gag in TV sitcoms than as a viable health therapy, but a good Avocado moisturizer mask really can help your skin.

The active ingredient in an Avocado's oil is Vitamin D which works to penetrate and nourish the skin, helping to rejuvenate it and encouraging new tissue growth, allowing the surface level of our epidermal cells to stay younger longer. So if your wife ever scared you in the middle of the night by plastering her face up in so much bright green Avocado oil that you woke up thinking a space alien was in bed with you; don't get mad! Because the benefits of this medicinal treatment, and all of the others mentioned in this chapter, far outweigh the discomfort!

Conclusion: Staying Healthy For Life

In the stress filled world of today, staying healthy can seem like a regular 9 to 5 job. The number one complaint for most of us is that we just don't have time to take care of our health. This is the reason why so many of us today would like to just pop a quick pill to get over whatever is bothering us. But unfortunately there is no quick fix when it comes to our health.

We need to break away from our preconceived and prepackaged notions and reintroduce ourselves to the resources that nature can provide. As we have learned in this book, herbal medicine has been with us for a long time, and it isn't going anywhere anytime soon. Everything we could ever need is right there in front of us, we just have to know how to take it. Once we do, healthy living and healing will not be far behind.

FREE Bonus Reminder

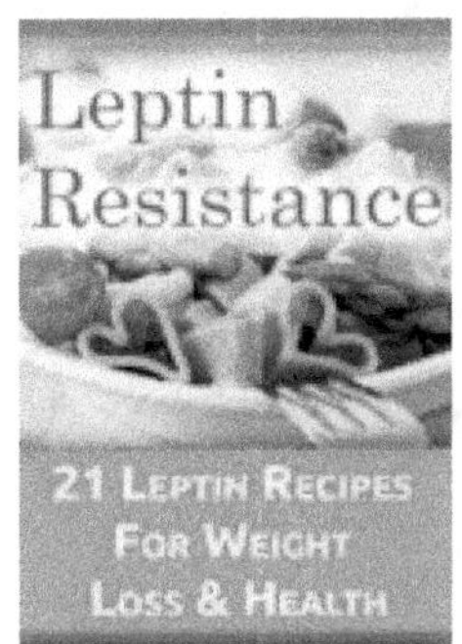

If you have not grabbed it yet, please go ahead and download your special bonus report *"Leptin Resistance. 21 Leptin Recipes For Weight Loss & Healthy Living"*.
Simply Click the Button Below

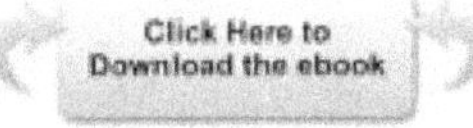

OR **Go to This Page**
http://easyweightlossway.com/free/

BONUS #2: More Free & Discounted Books
Do you want to receive more Free & Discounted Books?
We have a mailing list where we send out our new Books when they go free or with a discount on Kindle. Click on the link below to sign up for Free & Discount Book Promotions.
=> **Sign Up for Free & Discount Book Promotions** <=

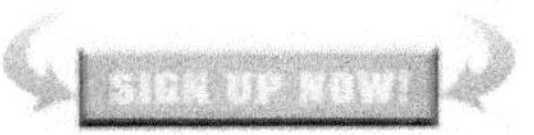

OR Go to this URL
http://zbit.ly/1WBb1Ek